# 21 LOSE WEIGHT: WINNING TIPS

## BEGIN A HEALTHFUL MINDSET AND LIFESTYLE CHANGE!

## Isobel McGrath

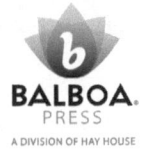

**BALBOA**
PRESS

A DIVISION OF HAY HOUSE

This book is a work of non-fiction. Unless otherwise noted, the author
and the publisher make no explicit guarantees as to the accuracy of
the information contained in this book and in some cases, names
of people and places have been altered to protect their privacy.

Balboa Press books may be ordered through booksellers or by contacting:

Balboa Press
A Division of Hay House
1663 Liberty Drive
Bloomington, IN 47403
www.balboapress.com
1 (877) 407-4847

Because of the dynamic nature of the Internet, any web addresses or
links contained in this book may have changed since publication and
may no longer be valid. The views expressed in this work are solely those
of the author and do not necessarily reflect the views of the publisher,
and the publisher hereby disclaims any responsibility for them.

The author of this book does not dispense medical advice or prescribe the use
of any technique as a form of treatment for physical, emotional, or medical
problems without the advice of a physician, either directly or indirectly. The
intent of the author is only to offer information of a general nature to help
you in your quest for emotional and spiritual well-being. In the event you use
any of the information in this book for yourself, which is your constitutional
right, the author and the publisher assume no responsibility for your actions.

Any people depicted in stock imagery provided by Thinkstock are
models, and such images are being used for illustrative purposes only.
Certain stock imagery © Thinkstock.

Print information available on the last page.

ISBN: 978-1-5043-9468-0 (sc)
ISBN: 978-1-5043-9469-7 (e)

Balboa Press rev. date: 01/30/2018

# DISCLAIMER

The information in this Book is not intended to be used as medical advice or treatment and prevention of any kind of disease. You must consult your physician prior to starting any nutrition, exercise or supplementation program since there may be risks for people in poor health, pre-existing physical and/or mental health conditions. This publication is intended for informational purposes only.

For information contact:
721 A1A Beach Boulevard,
Suite 7
St. Augustine, Florida, USA 32080

http://www.isobelmcgrath.com

# ACKNOWLEDGEMENTS

I wish to acknowledge the following people who have helped me on this journey. Especially Nancy Weston, my dream work partner for her continuous encouragement and expert editorial support.

I have so much admiration and gratitude for all the many people who have entrusted me with their life stories and allowed me to assist in their healing. As I have given, I have received and learned so much more in return. For this I am eternally grateful.

I'd like to acknowledge and thank all the people who have utilized my cd and mp3 programs throughout the years. I'd like to particularly thank the countless number of people who have called, and wrote just to tell me how much my work has helped them.

Last, but not least, I want to thank those clients of mine who kept asking me to write this book. Thank you for inspiring me and believing that this information can make a difference in others' lives.

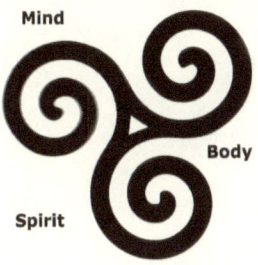

# DEDICATION

George Paul, who has encouraged my work and challenged my thinking for over twenty years. Thanks for always believing in me.

# CONTENTS

# INTRODUCTION

My intention is to inspire and motivate those who struggle and are unhappy with their weight. I am offering tips to help you make the change you desire. Most of the people who come to me already know about calories, nutrition and have been dieting on and off for years. They know what they should be doing and what they need to stop doing.

I am not a nutritionist, and this is not the focus of my work. My expertise is working with the mind. What I do know is that more and more, research acknowledges the detrimental effects of unnatural sugar on our moods and ability to think clearly, as well as on our waist line! The stomach/the gut is our second brain. If you want to feel less stressed it behooves you to eat as many natural foods as possible. Eating regularly and staying away from soda has made an enormous difference in client's lives.

I have collected these words of wisdom from my 22 years of experience in helping men and woman take control of their eating behavior. In no way am I implying that this is an easy task. But what I do know is the overwhelm people feel when they once again tackle losing weight. You are not alone. This is the natural cycle of change. You will slip, and get off track. It is my hope that these tips will help to ease the disappointment in yourself and give you the encouragement to persevere. When we feel overwhelmed, the only way forward is to break things down and start small, and master one thing before moving on to the next. Let's start over and begin again....

~ ~ ~ ~

# HOW TO USE THIS BOOK

Read through the whole book and choose the tips most relevant to you to be worked on later.

Read Tip 1 and 2 each morning to help you begin your day with a positive healthy mindset.

You can choose to practice one tip per day or one tip per week. Once you have mastered that tip you can move onto the next.

It is often best to start with the tip that is easiest first, then build on that by adding the next tip that is challenging for you. Be patient with yourself. It takes time to change habitual patterns. Change is not linear. Remember you are not a robot. As humans we are apt to go back and forth. Keep persevering.

# TIPS AT A GLANCE

1. Erase the word diet from your mind and vocabulary.
2. Think in terms of adopting a healthy lifestyle. Commit to healthful choices today.
3. Stop weighing yourself on the scale daily.
4. To increase your motivation, to lose weight dwell on the benefits of eating healthfully.
5. This is a learning period. Monitor and keep notes on what works, and what doesn't.
6. Stop destructive critical self-talk. Accept that you made an unhealthful choice(s) or you made a mistake. Mentally rehearse what you will do in the future.
7. Stop thinking in extremes: "You ate good or bad".
8. Aim for progress, doing better than previously. Know that we are all imperfect.
9. Think in terms of percentages. Be objective, "how did you do overall?" Give credit where it is due.
10. Keep a food journal. Write down what you plan on eating and the quantity, before you eat.
11. Eat only when you are hungry and eat before you are ravenous. If you are not hungry and crave food, address the underlying feelings.
12. If you are hungry think it through. Ask yourself, how will I feel after I have eaten this particular food I crave?
13. Do not shop when hungry. Write a grocery list and follow it. Buy healthy snacks. Being prepared makes it easier to eat healthily and lose weight.

14. Drink pure delicious water often. Stop confusing thirst for hunger.
15. Eat Mindfully. Take deep breaths, focus on the food, chew slowly and enjoy. Stop eating when you are comfortably satisfied.
16. Increase your physical activity as it speeds up your metabolism, burns calories and tones the body.
17. Reduce stress and you will stop emotional eating. Take deep belly breaths.
18. STOP when tempted. Refocus on your objective and plan for success.
19. Life balance is necessary, not optional.
20. Stop judging. Use the 4-step process – assess, accept, let go and feel empowered.
21. Stop making excuses. It is time to lovingly discipline your-self.

# DIETS DON'T WORK

## YOU ARE NOT ON A DIET . . .

Studies show 95% of diets fail and most will regain their lost weight in 1 to 5 years according to statistics on Weight Discrimination: A Waste of Talent, The Council on Size and Weight Discrimination. (Retrieved July 18, 2011, from http://www.cswd.org/index.html)

The word "diet" implies a short-term change. Focusing on losing weight is not enough. Research shows focusing on the overall health benefits of eating healthily and physical activity leads to long-term change and stops yoyo dieting.

Commit to your body's overall health on a daily basis and the weight will drop off as a result of this. This will create a change in your inner belief system. This is a deeper internal commitment to taking good care of your body, rather than an external fixation on losing weight and looking good.

Of course, looking and feeling good is important also,

but it is challenging to stay motivated and see the benefits daily. You can assess your eating choices, the consequences of these and your physical activity daily. This will help you stay focused on tangible results and help you see progress, even when the scale does not reflect the changes you have made. It can be extremely disheartening not to see your progress reflected back to you on the scale (see tip 16).

You are now adopting a healthy lifestyle to last a lifetime. You are adopting healthy eating behaviors to last a lifetime. This mindset will help you stay focused, encouraged and motivated daily, helping you lose weight and maintain the weight loss.

Being at a healthy weight is an ongoing goal which requires consistent attention. Just like when you are driving, you still need to check your surroundings, be mindful and know where you are going. Being aware of what you are thinking, about to eat, and the effect this food will have on your body becomes part of your daily routine.

Remember when you have a holiday or go on vacation, your body comes with you!

## REFLECTIONS

*How long have I been dieting?*

*What has the outcome been while using the dieting mindset?*

*What are my concerns if I stop dieting?*

*Do I accept that there is no short-term fix?*

*Am I willing to commit to taking care of my body for the rest of my life, beginning today?*

*Am I willing to give up the dieting mindset and focus on eating healthily for the benefits of my body, mind and spirit?*

- *If so, how will I be thinking differently today?*

- *How will I feel physically and psychologically if I shift my mindset to committing to my overall health and well-being rather than dieting?*

*What words of encouragement can I say to myself to help stay focused?*

*What actions will I be taking today?*

*Other notes to myself*

> **TIP 2: Think in terms of adopting a healthy lifestyle. Committing to healthy choices affects your body, mind and spirit today and in the future.**

# "YES!"

## I DO AND I WILL . . .

I vow, I make a solemn promise to myself *for* myself, from this day forth to take loving action to care for my mind, body and spirit.

We choose to invest in education to improve ourselves and to have a career. We choose a job to allow us financial freedom. We choose the place we live, the car we drive because it meets our needs and hopefully makes us happy. We make choices all the time to ensure our well-being and happiness. If you do not decide to do this with your health, what are the long-term consequences? For example, possible diabetes, high cholesterol, sore joints from carrying around extra weight, feeling unattractive, depression etc.

In order to make change, you need to make not only a decision but a **sincere commitment to yourself and your loved ones** to choose a healthy lifestyle. This commitment is very serious, just like a marriage, or when you sign a contract. You are giving your word that you will keep working on this. You will not give up on yourself. You expect challenges and will persevere. You know that the contract does not end. It is continual for the rest of your life. In order to stop yourself from being overwhelmed by the magnitude of this decision and the fear of failure, it is best to commit in small increments - one minute at a time, one hour and one day at a time.

## REFLECTIONS

*What thoughts, feelings and concerns do I have about making this commitment to take care of my body?*

*How do I feel about taking full responsibility for the choices I make?*

*What mind set will help me during challenging times so I will not give up on my commitment?*

*When I feel overwhelmed, can I give myself permission to commit to my health, one minute at a time, one hour at a time or one day at a time?*

*Am I willing to write a contract to care for my health today?*
*   *If not, explore why*

_Contract:_

For example: _I choose to commit to my health. I commit to making my health a top priority in my life today. I am willing to take full responsibility for what I feed my body, my physical activity and my stress level today._

I NOW choose to commit to .......


_Other notes to myself_

# STOP!

## IT IS BEST TO STOP WEIGHING YOURSELF DAILY . . .

If the weight reflected on the scale has the power to either make you happy or sad, then you need to stop being obsessed by the number on the scale. We can fluctuate so easily from day to day just from water retention alone.

If you find that weighing yourself is necessary and motivating for you, then weigh yourself once per week, remembering that fluctuations and stagnation are to be expected.

It is possible to gain weight as you become healthier. For example, becoming toned and building muscle weighs more than fat. It is possible to lose inches and not reduce your overall weight. If this occurs do not get discouraged, focus on the fact that you are healthier.

Weighing yourself is not necessary. You will feel the difference in your body and clothes and do not need the confirmation of the scale. Focus on the positive choices you are making, the increase in energy and the increase in your physical activity rather than solely on your weight.

## REFLECTIONS

*What happens when I weigh myself?*

- *What do I think?*

- *How do I feel and for how long?*

*Did I refrain from weighing myself today?*
- *If so, why?*

*Can I focus on the positive choices I am making, rather than solely on my weight?*

*What can I do to help myself to continue to focus on health and well-being?*

*Other notes to myself*

# Benefits

## FOCUS ON THE BENEFITS . . .

<u>Benefits of Losing Weight</u>

*I will have more energy.*
*I will feel lighter.*
*I will be free of possible health concerns.*
*I will feel more attractive and confident.*
*I will feel more in control.*
*I will feel proud of myself.*
*I will be able to travel with ease.*
*I will look great for my child's wedding.*
*I will be able to play with my grandchildren.*

If you are tempted to eat unhealthy foods, review the benefits of losing weight. Think it through. What are the consequences? Will you feel closer or further away from being healthy and slim?

The key to staying motivated is to focus on the benefits of a healthy lifestyle and losing weight. Focus on the positives. What is in it for you? What do you have to gain by losing weight? Imagine you are a sales person selling this image to you. The benefits are so overpowering that you fall in love with the healthier you and will do what it takes to get what you want. You need to convince yourself to readily give up the short-term gratification for the long-term benefits.

For example, you will have more energy, you will feel lighter, you will be free of possible health concerns, you will feel more attractive, be able to travel with ease, look great for your child's wedding, play with your grandchildren etc.

Do not focus on feelings of deprivation. Feeling sorry for yourself for what you are giving up is unhelpful and can cause you to rebel. Think to yourself that you have eaten this way for long enough. Been there done that! You know the consequences.

You now embrace maturity and it is time for a healthier lifestyle.

## REFLECTIONS

*What are the benefits of losing weight?*

- *How will I feel physically?*


- *How will I feel psychologically?*

*How often did I review these benefits today?*

*What can I do to help me remain focused on short and long-term benefits of adopting a healthy lifestyle?*

*What can I do to help me continue to think of the benefits of eating healthily and in moderation as opposed to focusing on feelings of deprivation?*

> **TIP 5: Treat this period as a learning period.**
> **Monitor and keep notes on what works,**
> **and what does not work for you.**

# LEARNING

## EXPERIMENT AND LEARN . . .

Experimenting & Learning: To eat healthily, drink water, and increase physical activity. What works? What was *not* helpful?

Know that as you make changes in your life style you will be going through a transition. During this time, it is important that you recognize that you are going through a learning process. You are learning what works for you. What helps? What does not help? Be open to learning, and experiment during this period. Know that change is uncomfortable; it is stressful, but necessary until more healthful habits are formed.

For example: Experiment with different healthful foods. For instance, instead of having a breakfast bar on the go, make a point to sit down and eat oatmeal with cinnamon, a boiled egg, or yogurt. Substitute veggies for chips, etc.

Evaluate the experience and the outcome. If you didn't like it, that's fine. If you experiment you may be pleasantly surprised that there are healthier alternatives that you *do* enjoy.

## REFLECTIONS

*I am committed to making change. What did I learn today?*

*What is helpful?*

*What is unhelpful?*

*What am I willing to experiment with in the future?*

# CREATE YOUR FUTURE

## FOCUS ON LEARNING FROM THE SITUATION . . .

Self-criticism keeps you locked into the current problem. Judgment shuts down creativity and problem-solving abilities.

> *There is a law in psychology that if you form a picture in your mind of what you would like to be, and you keep and hold that picture there long enough, you will soon become exactly as you have been thinking.*
> *- William James*

Ask yourself, "What could I have done differently?" Write down this alternative. Mentally rehearse the alternative behavior using all 5 senses. See, hear, smell, taste and feel your new behavior. If you mentally repeat this 3 times you are more likely to practice this alternative behavior in the future.

Vow to change your behavior and take positive

action from here on out. You can't rewrite the past. You can only write the present. So, put all your energy into letting go and starting over.

For example, in my town Tuesday is pizza special $7.99 a pie. Last Tuesday I bought 2 pies for the family. By myself I had 3 slices from it and regretted that choice immediately after devouring the last slice. (Feeling uncomfortable, guilty and regretful are all inner signals to assess your behavior and learn from it.) I therefore decided I will refrain from eating 3 slices in the future, 2 slices is sufficient. No matter how wonderful they taste, I will not be drawn into eating more than 2 slices. I'm now committed to eating in moderation.

## REFLECTIONS

*I now utilize positive self–talk: "I am in transition, set backs are completely normal. Berating myself is unhelpful. I focus my attention on learning from the situation."*

*What could I have done differently (thoughts and action)?*

*I now commit to this plan of action by writing down this alternative.*

*I now am locking this into my subconscious mind by mentally imagining and rehearsing the alternative behavior. **I will mentally rehearse this 3 times**. This way I will be more prepared and apt to behave differently in the future.*

> **What the mind can conceive, it can achieve!**
> **- Napoleon Hill**

# BLACK AND WHITE

## THINGS AREN'T BLACK AND WHITE . . .

Thinking, "I ate good or bad today" is black-and white, all-or-nothing thinking which is a cognitive distortion. When we find ourselves doing this, it is an indication that we are very emotional. For example, if you overeat, chances are you think, "That's it, I failed. I may as well give up". So, you continue making unhealthy choices for the rest of the day, perhaps for the rest of the week. You berate yourself. You feel guilty and bad, so you eat even more to escape these feelings. So the cycle continues.

When we find ourselves doing this, it is an indication that we are very emotional and need to utilize some stress management tools. Speak to yourself the way you would to a friend. Be compassionate. Everyone makes mistakes from time to time. Nobody eats perfectly all the time. Encourage yourself to let go of the past and start anew.

The sooner you stop berating yourself, the sooner you will get back on track.

## REFLECTIONS

*Did I think in terms of black or white, success or failure today?*

- *Did I recognize I was being overly emotional?*

- *Did I feel like a failure and gave up on trying?*

*What else was going on that could have contributed to feeling this way?*

*What can I do to let go of the situation and start over?*

*Positive self-talk may help: "I am in transition, set backs are completely normal. Berating myself is unhelpful. Everyone makes mistakes from time to time. Nobody eats perfectly all the time. I will encourage myself to let go of the past and start anew."*

*Other notes to myself*

# A IM FOR PROGRESS

## PLEASE STOP BERATING YOURSELF . . .

It is unhelpful. It actually perpetuates negative thoughts and feelings, which can lead to unhealthy choices and overeating. When you slip up and make an unhealthy choice. Start over, begin afresh.

Knowing that we are all humanly imperfect and aiming for progress not perfection, keeps your goals realistic and helps keep you encouraged to continue and to preserve.

Remember everyone slips and makes mistakes. However, it is those who persevere that are successful. This is why the 12 step programs use the slogan, "Progress not Perfection". Most set backs are caused by having expectations that are too high. It is best to set realistic goals which can be achieved.

Therefore, be aware of the tendency when emotional to think in extremes. Instead, think in terms of percentages, rather than classifying yourself as a failure (see Tip 9).

# REFLECTIONS

*Rate your achievements on a scale of 100% for today:*

### *Progress Rate*

*10%   20%   30%   40%   50%   60%   70%   80%   90%   100%*

_____ _____ _____ _____ _____ _____ _____ _____ _____ _____

*Did I drink water today?*

- *When?*

- *How much?*

*Did I do any physical activity (standing, walking, taking the stairs) today?*

- *When?*

- *How much?*

*Did I make any healthy choices today?*

- *Breakfast*

- *Snack*

- *Lunch*

- *Snack*

- *Dinner*

- *Snack*

*When were my portion sizes appropriate?*

*How do I feel about my progress today?*

*What will help me persevere?*

*Other notes to myself*

# Be fair

## BE OBJECTIVE . . .

How did you do overall? How were you doing before the slip? Give credit where it is due. Take into account any physical activity, how much water you drank, and the healthy choices you *did* make.

The truth is, very few people have perfect days of eating healthily. It is more helpful to think in terms of percentages. You are aiming for 100% that is, making healthy choices all day long. That is an A+ score. However, achieving a 50-70% is good. A 70 -80% is very good. An 80-95% is an A which is great. A+ 95-100% is excellent. That means you made healthy choices all day.

# REFLECTIONS

*Rate your achievements on a scale of 100% for today:*

**Progress Rate**

10%   20%   30%   40%   50%   60%   70%   80%   90%   100%

_____ _____ _____ _____ _____ _____ _____ _____ _____ _____

*Did I drink water today?*

- *When?*

- *How much?*

*Did I do any physical activity (standing, walking, climbing stairs) today?*

- *When?*

- *How much?*

*Did I make ANY healthy choices today?*

- *Breakfast*

- *Snack*

- *Lunch*

- *Snack*

- *Dinner*

- *Snack*

*When were my portion sizes appropriate?*

*How do I feel about my progress today?*

*What can I do to help persevere?*

*Other notes to myself*

# WRITE IT DOWN

## RECORDING YOUR CHOICES MAKES A DIFFERENCE...

Research shows that those who record their food intake lose more weight and stay on track than those who do not. As you record the food you eat, you become more conscious of the choices you are making. This improves your ability to think things through, rather than automatically reaching for food.

Most weight loss plans suggest recording after you eat. I propose that you do the opposite if you truly want to change your eating behavior. If you record before you eat, you will be fully aware of your intentions, the caloric content, and how your mind and body will feel afterwards.

Lots of clients tell me that mindless eating is their main downfall. For example, they find themselves finishing the bag of potato chips or cookies when they only intended to have a few.

Recording before you eat will help you create the mindset

necessary to make permanent lifestyle changes. Doing this will help you create the habit of thinking through your food choices. This awareness will afford you a little time, similar to hitting a pause button, so that you may reconsider your intentions. It is in this brief window of time that conscious choice begins.

It takes time and effort to create such a habit, so please be gentle with yourself and do not get discouraged. You are changing thought patterns and actions that have been around for a long time. There is no quick fix. This takes commitment, consistency and courage to be honest with yourself.

Some clients choose to take a photograph of the food they are considering eating. Again, this buys you a little time to pause and reconsider. At the end of the day they review the times they succumbed and the times they reframed from giving in to their urges.

If you fail to record *prior* to eating, you can record midway through or after you finish. Recording and reviewing your actions after each meal is extremely important and beneficial in creating new neural pathways of conscious, responsible awareness of your eating behavior. This is necessary in order to achieve long-term success.

When you record every meal, please also rate your **hunger level** and your **stress level** on a scale of 1 to 10, where 1 is not at all, 5 is moderate and 10 is at the highest. If you find yourself overindulging etc., journal about your feelings and what led up to those choices. Adopt a mindset of curiosity and a willingness to learn from these situations.

Level (1-10)

Hunger _____ Stress _____ Food _____ Portion _____ Beverage _____ Outcome _____

# REFLECTIONS

*On a scale of 1 to 10, where 1 is not at all, 5 is moderate and 10 is at the highest.*

*How hungry are you?*

*How stressed are you?*

*What did you eat (You can take a photograph and ask yourself would you be comfortable sharing this photograph)?*

*What did you drink?*

*How were your portion  sizes?*

*Did I record this before, during, or after I ate?*

*Did I do this for everything I ate?*

- *If not, why not?*

*Other notes to myself*

> **TIP 11: Eat only when you are hungry and eat before you are ravenous. If you are not hungry and crave food, address the underlying feelings.**

# GOOD QUESTIONS

## ARE YOU *REALLY* HUNGRY?

Before you go to eat, focus on your abdomen, not your head or the clock. Tune into your stomach and ask yourself, "On a scale of 1 to 10, 1 being not hungry and 10 being famished, am I hungry?" If so, rate your hunger.

If you are not hungry, then ask yourself, "Why am I seeking food?" Become curious and investigate. Remember you can feel more than one feeling at the same time, we are multifaceted human beings. Are you feeling emotional, tired, lonely, bored, sad, angry, stressed? If so, then tend to those feelings.

Eating is only a short-term fix. There is no point in berating or criticizing yourself. Tend to your feelings by acknowledging them. Remember feelings are not facts. They are often irrational. Learn to validate your feelings. For example, say to yourself, "yes, it has been a tough day." "Yes, you do feel lonely." Be your own best friend and listen to your feelings. You may choose to journal about your feelings. As you write down how you feel, you can release the feelings.

Finally, ask yourself, if there is something you can do (besides eating) to help you feel better. For example, calling a friend, taking a shower or bath, reading, deep breathing, going to bed early. By acknowledging your feelings and taking loving action to tend to those feelings you are taking care of your entire being - mind, body and spirit.

Food is a way in which we self-medicate. Once you attend to your feelings there is no need to reach for food or an alcoholic drink as a quick fix. Emotions come and go, like the waves of the ocean, but they need to be acknowledged, in order to dissipate.

To review, ask yourself, "How hungry am I?" Rate your hunger on a scale of 1 to 10 (1 being not hungry, 10 being famished).

If you are not hungry, you do not NEED to eat. Investigate how you are truly feeling, and attend to that feeling. For example, if you are tired or stressed, pause, take a few deep breaths. As you exhale repeat the word "RELAX." Remind yourself, "Feelings come and go, this too shall pass".


## REFLECTIONS

*Why am I thinking about food, or seeking food right now?*

*Am I hungry? If so, rate your hunger on a scale of 1 to 10 (1 being not hungry, 10 being famished).*

*If I am hungry (rated 4 to 10) I will make healthy choices that will lead me closer to my goals.*

*If I am not hungry (rated 1 to 3), what am I feeling? Journal as to what thoughts are causing these feelings.*

- *Stressed?*
- *Tired?*
- *Bored?*
- *Lonely?*
- *Angry?*
- *Confused?*
- *Sad?*
- *Upset?*
- *Hurt?*
- *Tempted?*
- *Deprived?*
- *Deserving?*
- *Joyful?*
- *Happy?*

VALIDATE: It is okay that I feel this way. I am willing to give myself compassion and talk to myself kindly as I would do to my best friend or loved one.

*I would say ....*

_____

_____

_____

ACTION: What can I do to feel better?

_____

What has helped in the past?

_____

_____

Would it help to call a supportive friend, take a shower or bath, read, deep breathe, walk, stretch, or go to bed early?

_____

_____

What I truly need instead of food is kindness from myself right now. I can take healthy action on my behalf, such as ...

_____

_____

_____

_____

_____

_____

*Other notes to myself*

# THINK IT THROUGH

## WILL THIS HELP?

Ask yourself, "Will this help me lose weight?" Think of the consequences. Choose food that will energize you and make you feel good about your choices. Make healthful choices which will make you feel good physically and mentally.

If you rate your hunger between 8 and 10, be alert. Eat slowly. When we are very hungry we have less control over our eating behavior. It is best to eat before you are ravenous.

If you decide to have a treat or unhealthful food, then decide on the portion size beforehand. Eat in moderation.

> *Wisdom consists in the anticipation of consequences.*
> *- Norman Cousins*

Your mindset is extremely important. Give yourself the permission to enjoy this food. Slow down, be mindful and savor each mouthful. Assess afterwards, did this taste as good as you imagined it to be? Could you have eaten less and been satisfied?

## REFLECTIONS

*Affirm: "Before I eat, let me pause and think through the consequences of my choices".*

*How will I feel after I have eaten this particular food I crave?*

*How will I feel physically and mentally immediately after I have eaten this particular food I crave?*

*How will I feel physically and mentally in the long term?*

*Will I be critical of myself?*

*Will this help me be healthy and lose weight?*

*Do I feel in control of my choice and portion size?*

*How hungry am I on a scale of 1 to 10? (1 being not hungry, 10 being famished).*

*How does my hunger level affect my ability to remain in control of my choices i.e. my ability to think through the long-term consequences?*

*Other notes to myself*

**TIP 13: Do not shop when hungry. Write a grocery list and follow it. Buy healthy snacks. Being prepared makes it easier to eat healthfully and lose weight.**

# PREPARE

## PREPARATION IS KEY . . .

You need to make healthful choices easy and convenient for you. So many people slip up because they are expecting way too much of themselves. They expect to be cooking fresh meals at home every night etc.

Focus on harm reduction, rather than how you would choose to eat in a perfect world, when you had all the time you wanted and needed to prepare meals.

You need to make things as easy for you as possible and you need to have healthy foods available. Nowadays, they sell apples and vegetables in the grocery store that are already peeled and cut up. Yes, they may be more expensive, but if you find yourself too busy to peel fruit or vegetables it is worth paying extra for the convenience. When you are in the habit of eating healthfully, you can take more time for yourself to prepare healthful meals.

Going to the grocery store less frequently and with a list of what you need for the week will help you be less tempted to pick up unhealthful foods. It's important to buy healthful snacks that you can take with you when you are in a hurry. Having healthful snacks readily available will make it easier for you to follow a healthy lifestyle.

Choose to eat foods that are as close to their natural state as possible. This will ensure you are getting the best nutrition possible. Think of those foods as the best options, then in terms of foods that are moderately healthy and finally foods that are the least healthy. Aim to eat rarely from the least healthy category.

Make a list of easy healthful snacks, breakfasts, lunches and dinners. Put the list on the refrigerator and in your cell/mobile phone. Consult your list regularly as it will make food choices much less stressful and easier to implement.

## REFLECTIONS

*List of breakfasts*

*List of lunches*

*List of dinners*

*Easy healthful snacks*

*Other notes to myself*

# Water, Water

## THE BODY NEEDS WATER . . .

The body is predominantly made up of water. It needs pure water to flush out the kidneys, rid the body of toxins, and for a healthy complexion.

> *Drinking water is like washing out your insides. The water will cleanse the system, fill you up, decrease your caloric load and improve the function of all your tissues.*
> *- Kevin R. Stone*

Often people confuse hunger for thirst. To prevent this confusion, get into the habit of filling up on water. The easiest way my clients and myself have found to do this is to drink a glass of water first thing in the morning and before eating. It is easy to pair drinking a glass of water before breakfast, lunch, snacks and dinner.

You can drink herbal decaffeinated teas, and add lemon

or cucumber to water for natural flavoring. Remember to drink the recommended 8 glasses of water per day.

## REFLECTIONS

*What is my caffeine intake?*

*How does caffeine affect my thinking and my body?*

*How much water did I drink today?*

*How can I improve my water intake?*

*Other notes to myself*

> **TIP 15: Eat mindfully. Take deep breaths, focus on the food, chew slowly and enjoy. Stop all outside distractions. Stop eating when you are comfortably satisfied.**

# FOCUS

## FOCUS YOUR FULL ATTENTION WHEN EATING . . .

Slow down and enjoy the experience of eating. Begin with taking a few deep breaths. Stop the mental chatter. Think of all that had to occur to bring this food to you – the sunlight, the crops, the farmers etc. This will help you create a positive mindset of gratitude.

Set the intention to be grateful for the food you are about to eat and that this food will nourish your mind, body and spirit.

Focus on the smell, texture and flavor of the food you are eating. Think about all that had to occur to bring this food to you. Chew your food slowly. Chewing aids digestion. Take your time, savor the experience.

People often tell me that they are too busy to sit down and just eat, so they approach eating as something they must get through quickly, so they can accomplish more.

This approach causes stress and increases indigestion. If you find yourself rushing, please time yourself to see how long this experience truly takes. Ask yourself: are you in a race with time? If so, you need to address this core issue as it often sabotages a healthful mindset and lifestyle.

## REFLECTIONS

*Did I remember to pause, take deep breaths to slow down, and focus before eating?*

*Did I set my intention to be grateful for the food I am about to eat?*

*Did I set the intention that my mind, body and spirit would be nourished?*

*Did I eat mindfully, by paying full attention to smell, texture and flavor of the food?*

*Did I take my time, chew slowly and savor the experience?*

*What challenges did I encounter?*

*What can I do to make progress next time?*

*Other notes to myself*

# ON THE MOVE

## PHYSICAL ACTIVITY MATTERS . . .

I often hear people say they dislike exercising, for a multitude of reasons. For some people exercising seems too high of a goal to achieve. That's understandable if you have had a negative history with exercising.

Start where you are at right now. Focus on increasing your physical activity. For example, take the stairs rather than the elevator. Park the car further away so you have further to walk. Get up and stretch often. Put hand weights next to your chair and when you watch TV, do some reps.

If you set small goals, that will help you get started. Aim for a 5-minute walk daily and then increase it to 10 minutes. Keep gently challenging yourself.

We often get bored with the same old routines, so experiment with different activities without putting pressure on yourself to make a commitment. As long as you are moving, you are doing well. All physical activity counts, so that 10-minute walk while you were on the phone was better than you sitting and chatting.

People are more consistent when they have a buddy to do physical activities with. Perhaps, to begin with you can ask a neighbor or friend if they would like to walk with you.

Clients who have wanted to exercise have benefited from having a personal trainer, belonging to a small workout group, and attending a regular exercise class.

## REFLECTIONS

*What physical activity did I do today?*

- *Walking*

- *Standing*

- *Biking*

- *Climbing the stairs*

- *Stretching*

- *Lifting*

- *A fitness class*

*Are there any fun ways in which I can increase my physical activity?*

*Did I set small achievable goals or were my goals too high?*

*Other notes to myself*

> **TIP 17: Reduce stress and you will stop emotional eating.**

# TAKE IT EASY

## TAKE A DEEP BREATH . . .

Stress increases cortisol levels and leads to weight gain. Most people are overwhelmed by the demands of life. Take a step back and assess the way in which you chose to live your life. If you cannot change external stressors, then change the way in which you view the things you consider stressful. For example, the children can be stressful, but they can also bring you joy.

Counseling and coaching can help you change the way you cope with stress. The easiest form of stress reduction I have found is **deep belly breathing**. You can do it with your eyes open or closed, standing or sitting.

Breathe in slowly through your nose for a count of 4. The air going into your nose should move downward so that you can feel your stomach rise. Breathe out though your mouth as your stomach naturally relaxes, to a count of 8.

Although the frequency of this breathing exercise will vary according to your health, the sequence is often done three times when you're beginning. Most people can work up to 5 to 10 minutes one to four times a day. The beauty of this exercise is that you can do it anywhere anytime. So, it is easily incorporated into your busy life. You can do it while standing in line, stopped at a stop light, before you answer the phone and before you choose to eat.

If you feel lightheaded at any time, discontinue the breathing exercise and continue your normal breathing.

## REFLECTIONS

*What efforts did I make to reduce stress today?*

*Did I take any deep belly breaths?*

*How can I remember to de-stress and increase the frequency of belly breathing?*

*Other notes to myself*

> **TIP 18: STOP when tempted. Refocus on your objective and plan for success.**

# STOP!

## THINK FIRST . . .

According to cognitive behavioral theory, it is not the events in life that upset us but the thoughts we think about those events that cause us to feel upset. This helps us understand why two people experiencing the same experience can have different reactions. For example, taking the same flight on an airplane: one person feels excited while the other is fearful. Therefore, if we want to change how we feel, we need to dispute our thoughts and beliefs, rather than accepting them as truth.

"STOP" is a cognitive behavioral tool that can help to improve impulse control and cope with stress. First, think or imagine a big red stop sign. If you were driving, you would not hesitate to stop in case of an accident. The same is true if you continue to be stressed. Your blood pressure and heart rate increases, increasing your risk of a heart attack.

Therefore, it is important to stay calm no matter what is happening in your life. Also, by remaining calm you have a better chance of clear and rational thinking, which will help you cope with the situation more effectively.

STOP is an acronym for Sensing, Thinking, Objective and Plan. If you are tempted to eat impulsively, stop immediately and ask yourself:

What am I **S**ensing/Feeling?

What am I **T**hinking?

What is my **O**bjective? (Hopefully, to stay calm, eat healthily and lose weight)

What is my **P**lan, given my objective?

For example, I am at the supermarket and feel tempted to buy a bar of chocolate.

I choose to **STOP** immediately and investigate.

-    What am I **S**ensing/Feeling?

     *"I am frustrated and tired"*

-    What am I **T**hinking?

     *"I deserve a treat, chocolate will give me the energy I need to get through the afternoon"*

-    What is my **O**bjective?

     *"My objective is to stay calm, eat healthily and lose weight"*

-    What is my **P**lan, given my objective?

I now dispute my original thoughts and utilize positive self-talk:

"I am okay, everyone gets frustrated from time to time. Eating chocolate will give me a boost of energy and then I will crash. I can eat an alternative healthier food that will sustain my energy. Let me take a few deep breaths and consciously choose to let this urge go. I feel happy with myself when I make healthier choices."

## REFLECTIONS

*How and when would I benefit from using the STOP sign tool?*

*Let me experiment with practicing the STOP sign tool (Sensing, Thinking, Objective and Plan):*

*What am I Sensing/Feeling?*

*What am I Thinking?*

*What is my Objective? (Hopefully, to stay calm, eat healthily and lose weight)*

*What is my Plan, given my objective?*

*What can I do to help acquire the habit of Stopping when tempted, refocusing on my objective, and making a plan for success?*

# BALANCE

## YOU COUNT . . .

I hear people say, "I don't have time for that." Yet we all know we make time for the things that are important to us. Studies verify that balance is paramount to our well-being. Yet women are notorious for putting themselves last on the list. You lead by example. By doing this you are silently teaching others that you are not as important as they are. This can lead to resentment on your part.

All too often, client's report food being their main source of pleasure and enjoyment. A chocolate bar becomes their treat for having worked all day etc. Or they are bored in the evening and find comfort from food in the kitchen cabinet. If food has become your main source of comfort and pleasure, then it is truly time to take stock of your emotional needs and formulate a plan of action as to how you can address these in a healthy manner.

It is time to stop self-sacrificing behaviors and to balance your life with creativity and play time. It is important to do things you enjoy. You will smile more and feel happier, which will positively impact everyone in your life.

Ask yourself, "What can I do daily or weekly to increase feelings of joy?

## REFLECTIONS

*Is my life out of balance? If so, in what ways?*

*Did I smile today?*

*Did I laugh today?*

*How can I increase my feelings of joy?*

*Do I have time for self-care, creativity and play?*

*If I gave myself permission to put my needs first, what would that look like?*

*What obstacles and are in my way?*

*Are there any small steps I can take to improve my life situation and my well-being?*

# JUDGE NOT

## ASSESS, DON'T JUDGE!

Ever wondered why all spiritual traditions teach "Judge not?" It so happens that research is in agreement with this.

> *Letting go does not mean you agree or condone the behavior. Letting go simply means that you no longer choose to hold onto the feelings and live in the past. You choose to focus your thoughts, feelings and enthusiasm in creating the life you want. – Isobel McGrath*

If you want to be able to break out of old habitual ways of reacting, it is best to *assess* your behavior, rather than judge.

For example, you are out for dinner and you have the "death-by-chocolate" dessert. You judge yourself harshly, saying "What is wrong with me? My cholesterol is high, I'm going to die of a heart attack". Because you are so caught up in berating yourself, you run the risk of having a nightcap or cookies. You are not in the here and now. You are stuck in the past judging yourself for over-indulging.

Alternatively, you eat the "death-by-chocolate" dessert and you assess your behavior. You tell yourself, "I need to slow down and pay more attention when I'm dining out as I get so tempted by the desserts". In this situation, all of your focus goes into correcting your behavior and being more mindful of what you are doing now, rather than the past. So, you assess your behavior, learn from the consequences and move on.

By judging you run the risk of imprisoning yourself in a continuous cycle of anger, frustration, and apathy. These emotions are not only incapacitating, (you feel like giving up, what's the point in trying to do things differently when you continually fail) but can lead to physical illness.

Research in neuroscience shows that when we are stressed, which happens when we judge ourselves, a hormone called *norepinephrine* is released, which inhibits the brain's ability to constructively resolve stressful challenges and creatively problem solve. Thus, we fall back on habitual patterns i.e. we use old ways of coping.

How many times have you promised yourself that you would not light up that cigarette, have an alcoholic drink, reach for the cookie, or raise your voice at your spouse or children, or procrastinate? Yet, you find yourself doing it time and time again.

This may be due to the fact that judgment paralyzed your creativity and hindered your ability to act in new and constructive ways. So, judgment can hinder your ability to make progress.

Can we simply stop being judgmental? Firmly

established patterns of behavior require more than insight and understanding to be transformed.

The first step to changing your behavior is to gently acknowledge and accept this part of yourself that judges. The more you accept and forgive this part of yourself that has the tendency to judge, the easier it will be for you to notice this behavior and eventually you will become so skillful at noticing and observing yourself, that the time will come when you will be able to catch yourself *before* judging. So, eventually with practice, your impulse to judge will decrease and eventually disappear.

### 4 Steps to Assess, Accept, Learn, Let it go, to feel motivated and empowered to behave differently.

1. Witness and observe yourself judging with loving acceptance. Remember you are human and we all judge. Forgive yourself.

2. When you catch yourself say, "Here I go again, judging." Feel good about your progress in noticing yourself judging.

3. It is now your choice whether you continue in the cycle of judging. Choose to stop judging and learn to assess the situation. What would you prefer to happen? Do you have any control over this?

4. Accept the situation. Learn from the experience. Let it go and channel all your energy into moving forward with the attitude and behavior you now prefer. This increases your chances of persevering. Pick yourself up, dust yourself off and soldier on.

# REFLECTIONS

*When did I judge myself today?*

*Did I stop myself at any time and practice the 4 steps?*

*How can I remember to stop judging myself, assess my behavior, accept the past, and let go with the intention of behaving differently in the future?*

*Am I now willing to choose to let go of negative feelings about past behavior, learn from it and move forward?*

- *If not, why not?*

# BEGIN TODAY

## GET STARTED . . .

Stop being too lenient with yourself. There are no quick
fixes when it comes to permanent weight loss. There will
never be a perfect time to start. Life is messy, so accept this
and start with one small change. Every little action makes
a difference. It will help you build momentum, so you can
build on your successes.

Tomorrow never comes, all we have is the present. That
is why it is called a gift...the gift of life. So please start today
and take better care of your mind and body by feeding
yourself healthful nutritious food and beverages. As you
adopt a healthy lifestyle you will reap the benefits. Your body
will reward you for it, by granting you a longer, healthier life.

# REFLECTIONS

*How do I feel about being self-disciplined and responsible for my life choices?*

*Do I tend to be too tough or too lenient with myself?*

*What commitments did I follow through with today?*

*Did I choose not to follow through with anything today that I had committed to?*

- *If so, why?*

- *Was this in my best interest?*

*What can I say and do to stop myself from making excuses in the future?*

*Other notes to myself*

# FINAL THOUGHTS

Living a healthy lifestyle is a continuous journey that never ends. People have unrealistic expectations and expect to fully master their eating, as if we are robots!

We are human beings. We are complex and constantly in the flux of change; for example, every day we grow a little older. Life continually challenges us. We have emotional ups and downs.

So, in the midst of life, we continue to keep our stability and sense of control by choosing healthful foods and physical activities because we know these behaviors will help us think more clearly, which will help us cope with life with less stress and perhaps live a little longer.

I wish you happiness on your journey.

# ISOBEL MCGRATH PROGRAMS

Online Programs, CDS and MP3s:
Weight Loss
Smoking Cessation
Alcohol Cessation
Decrease Stress & Anxiety
Increase Self-Esteem & Confidence
Sleep Deeply Throughout the Night
Overcome Fear of Flying
Break Free of Co-dependency

**ALL OF THESE ARE AVAILABLE AT
WWW.ISOBELMCGRATH.COM**

# SPECIAL FREE OFFER

If you'd like to receive a **COMPLIMENTARY** mind makeover with 4 powerful guided exercises to help you feel calm and in control, or receive personal coaching, please visit www.IsobelMcGrath.com

To connect with Isobel, visit her on Facebook at www.facebook.com/IsobelMcGrathLLC or on her website at www.IsobelMcGrath.com and join the community of Isobel's blog and newsletter readers!

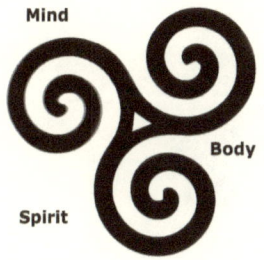